"Ever since I hpounds and build a and defined body, my the age of 50 has skyrocketed, making it necessary for me to develop a new workout plan specifically designed to keep my elderly clients healthy and in shape.

Over the past year, I came up with a system of simplified workouts which combine dynamic movements as well as concentrated actions, in order to keep my clients safe from injury and in constant development of muscle, and the workout plan has proven surprisingly effective.

As the number of clients I can work with is limited, I created and at-home version of that workout routine, which really only changes a couple of exercises with efficient alternatives, making it highly accessible for anyone to train and get in the best shape of their life regardless of age.

In the book, we are going to be discussing some of the basics about fitness that I always teach my clients about, in order for them to know why we are doing certain things, and then we will be shifting out focus to the key exercises of the routine, as well as adequate nutrition before heading into the structured workout plan.

With this information anyone can build an incredible body at home or at the gym, completely ignoring the side-effects of aging.

This being said, I welcome each and every one of you to my workout program, and I certainly hope we will be seeing amazing results together!"

Table of contents

Foreword 6
How do we grow our muscles? 8
The 3 Keys of Fitness 20
Training 21
      Push Day 29
      Pull day 43
      Leg Day 54
      Abs and Cardio 60
Nutrition 70
The Basics 74
      Getting started 99
Rest 108
Training plan 109
Weekly schedule 118

Foreword

The last thing before getting started will be mentioning that the workout program you are about to be mastering and the information that strongly ties to it have all been perfected in a personal trainer-client relationship environment, and the intensity of the workouts was adapted based on the joint and muscle capacities of each individual client.

For that matter, since you will be going unsupervised, we highly suggest paying additional attention to what your ligaments and muscles can handle in the beginning.

If an exercise is too difficult to complete in 4 sets and 12 repetitions, do as many repetitions as you can handle. That is more than sufficient to cause the tissue rupture required for muscle growth, while injury will only result in a delay in workouts and long-term results.

Now, to start our journey with the most important things to know when training, what are we really chasing? Muscle growth, as weight loss comes with it in this system. And how do we achieve muscle growth?

We'll find out starting with the next page…

How do we grow our muscles?

The simple answer people give is "training", but that is insufficient for us to completely understand the muscle building process...

At birth, our bodies have a certain amount of muscle fibers, all of them making up certain muscles, combined with ligaments creating the muscular system. Through the contraction and relaxation of your muscles, movement is achieved, when the brain signals the neuro-transmitters in your body to do a certain movement.

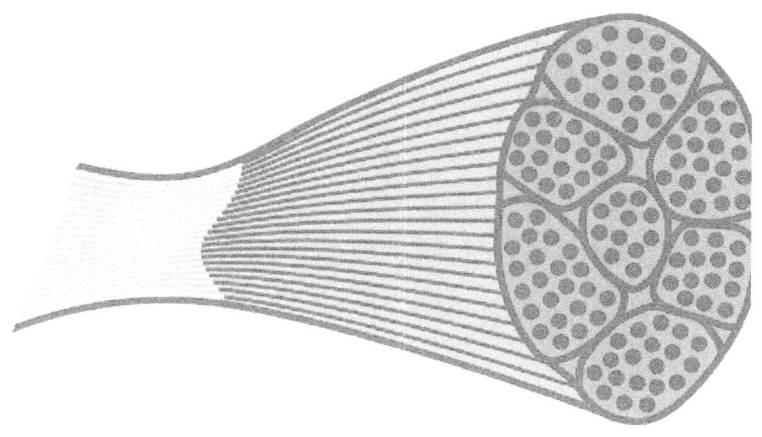

As we grow and develop, so do our muscles, becoming bigger and stronger, in order to support and motorize a bigger and heavier body. Usually this process continues until the muscles are strong enough to support our full-grown bodies, depending on the lifestyle we're living, the process may result in a thicker musculature in athletic individuals on specific parts of the body, and thinner muscles for the individuals who did not show signs of high physical activity during their growth period. The muscles we're left with naturally are not the limit however, not by a longshot, as mother-nature created us to be the most advanced living mechanisms, like other species, we also have the instinct of adaptation. Like our ancestors' bodies started to shed body-hair as the climate was warming up and adaptation was required to keep the body cool, the modern human can adapt to new situations just as well as his ancestors.

At the core of muscle growth stands the concept of adaptation, as our body is facing new challenges, such as lifting a weight that's too heavy, the ancient instinct of adaptation powers up and receives the message "We need to lift this but we are not strong enough, we need to adapt to heavier weights." and the muscle gaining process is let loose. This description is very primitive, as the process is a lot more complex, and we will get into details soon. After the need for adaptation is established, we need to provide stimulus in order to make the muscles grow, which is training. By constantly facing our bodies with new challenges, each time harder, the need for adaptation becomes a solid routine and the systems required to achieve muscle growth are given continuous work. If you've ever heard that consistency is the base of any fitness routine, now you know why, as the continuous stimulus is necessary to keep the body fired up and ready to develop.

Not all stimulus was created equal, and simply living, as in doing an everyday routine and activity will get your body to adapt only as much as needed, which has most likely been achieved by now, and the lack of further stimulus will have your body breaking down the muscle you already have, in order to reduce the amount of energy needed maintaining them, without actually using the power they generate for anything. The stimulus provided has to be hard enough to engage the muscle to a point where it can no longer complete the task, such as lifting the same weight 20 times, most likely for the 20th repetition your muscles will have exhausted.

When our muscles are exposed to sufficient stress, through the engagement in activities that are too difficult for our muscles to complete, such as lifting a 15 kg dumbbell using your bicep, the muscle gets damaged, with microscopic ruptures in the muscle fiber.

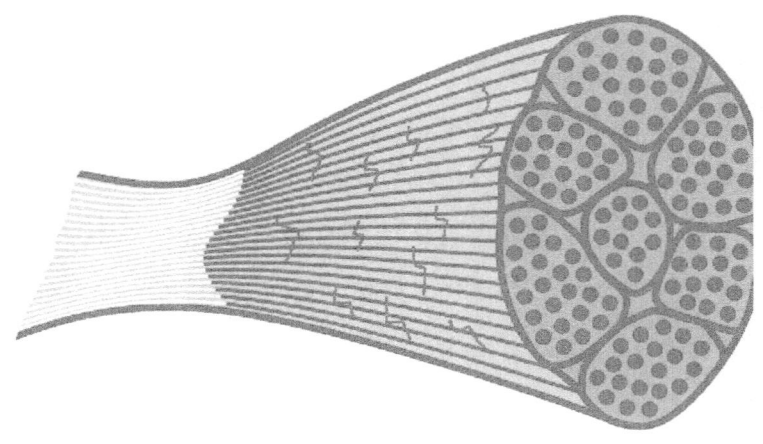

Believe it or not, this is exactly what bodybuilders train for, to damage their muscle fibers. It may sound counter intuitive how people interested in growing their muscles, are actually doing so with an activity that damages them. Science backs up their actions, as the damaging of the muscle fibers triggers a reaction through which cytokines, small molecules that help with muscle growth, which engage the immune system to repair the damaged fibers.

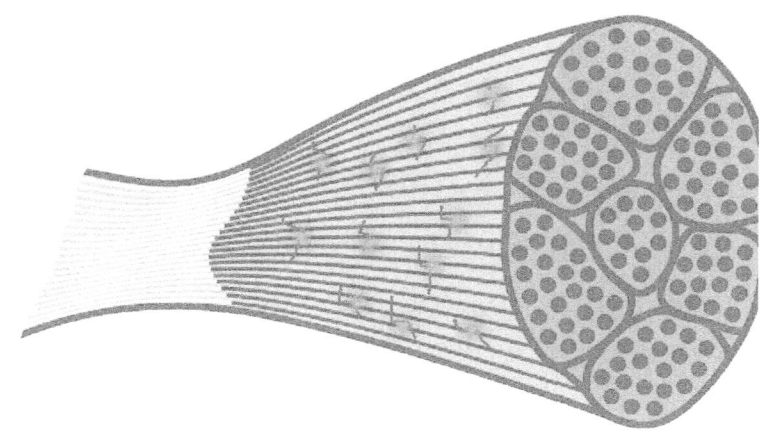

It is this very process that stimulates muscle growth, as the body is aware of the need for adaptation, the damaged muscle fibers are not only getting repaired, but this time, the body, if provided with the required materials, rebuilds the fibers bigger and stronger, eventually thickening the muscle.

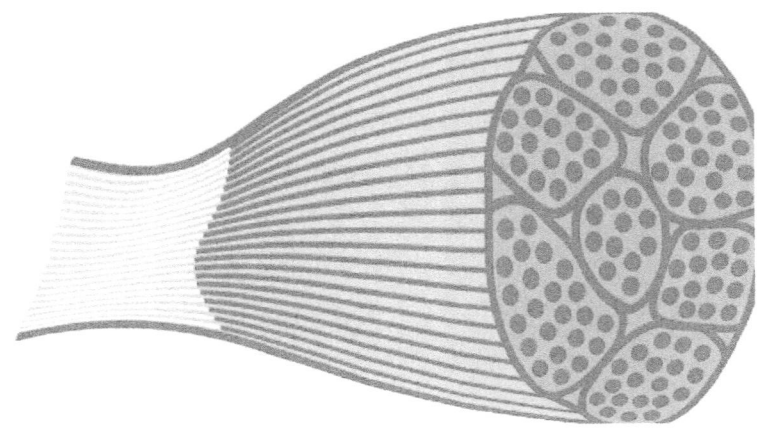

The bodybuilding community has been asking if there is a way to actually build *more* muscle fibers, which science quickly answered by saying no, the amount of muscle fibers we have are the same we did when we were born, and the only way to grow our muscles is by thickening the fibers, as increasing their number is impossible. The more often and intensely we damage the muscle fibers, the more intensely and often our body has to repair that damage, eventually turning this cycle into a routine.

Another key factor is what the fitness community calls "progressive overload", which in itself refers to the continuous increase of the workout intensity, in order to stimulate greater muscle growth. The reason behind it is once again purely scientific and logical, since our bodies have been adapting to the workouts since the first day, building bigger and stronger muscles in order to ensure progress, the weights or repetitions we started with are not as challenging as they were the first day, meaning we need to increase either the weights or the number of times we put our muscles under tension in order to provide the fibers with new cellular level tears, so the immune system can continue further building the muscle. This process of exposing the muscles to heavier stress and resistance, is called hypertrophy, a term we'll be using quite often.

Training is not the only essential element when it comes to building muscle, as our body cannot just repair the damaged tissue by itself, we need to provide it with the equivalent of raw building material, protein. The consumption of protein contributes to muscle maintenance, as well as muscle growth, as protein is broken down into the equivalent of building bricks, amino acids. Amino acids are used by the immune system in order to repair the damaged fiber into a bigger and stronger muscle, but we are responsible with providing the body with protein in order to be broken down and transformed into the priceless amino acids. We will cover nutrition in greater detail soon, giving a scientific approach, but for now we will move on to our third key element when it comes to muscle growth, rest.

The same way animals need rest in order to get their energy levels back up, so do humans, but at a cellular level, things are not as different. Our bodies need time to recover, while muscles can get fixed during the day, the best time for muscles to regenerate is during sleep, as the body slows down most of its functions, and can focus on the muscle fiber repair with more exclusivity. Imagine this process the same way a computer updates its operation system at night or after a restart, as during the day it is in use, with many processes running in the background, while at night or after a restart, the amount of tasks running is significantly lower, dedicating more resources towards an OS update.

This pretty much answers the question "What makes muscles grow?" in a nutshell, now we will be taking a look at each element in particular and the way to apply them towards building yourself a physique worthy of a Greek god.

With age, this process, as well as many others lose efficiency, and muscle gain won't be as easy as it is for a 20 year old young man who basically breathes testosterone and is in peak health condition.

This doesn't mean that muscle gain is impossible by any means, it is indeed very much possible and simple to achieve, but the quantity of muscle gained over a period of time will not match the quantity gained by a youngster over that same time, with the same training plan.

The 3 Keys of Fitness

These three elements make up the so called "keys" of fitness, needing all three of them in order for any healthy and exercise system to work, excluding one will only get you little to no progress. This is indeed a program that allows for very quick results, if respected, but long-term effects will require dedication and turning fitness into your lifestyle instead of having it be a solution for a problem. In the following we will go through all three elements, Training, Nutrition and Rest, bringing you both the basic knowledge, as well as the revolutionary techniques in all three domains in order to maximize results. First off, we have the fun part of building a Greek god-like body, Training.

Training

Training the muscular system is the first and most important step in the muscle-building process, as is stimulates the body to transform into a bigger, stronger and more functional mechanism. An effective training program is essential in order to see results, but with the fitness industry growing exponentially in the past 30 years, new diets, workout programs, supplements and ideologies appear almost on a daily basis, so before talking about your workout program, we need to further dissect what we know for sure about training, and build up from there. Different forms of training such as classic bodybuilding, calisthenics, crossfit, functional group classes, etcetera became endlessly competitive against each other, with the growing demand for body-defining activities, the market grew as well, and even though all forms of physical exercise are effective in one way or another, the adepts of different types of training started a propaganda against the others, spawning a vicious fight over the market.

We come to ask ourselves, what is the BEST form of physical exercise after all? In my opinion this is a question without answer, as each type has its advantages and disadvantages, and ultimately with the correct dedication and consistency, all forms will bring solid results, but in order to give a more specific perspective of how this workout plan found in this book was created, let's take a look at the basic principles involved.

- First and foremost, I started my fitness journey with bodybuilding, or to give you a more in depth answer, when I was 16 my parents got me a gym membership with a personal trainer, as my body was not exactly "manly", and it didn't seem like it was going to be anytime soon, unless I started doing some serious work in that matter. Bodybuilding is incredibly effective, as the primary goal of each exercise is to build size, by isolating the muscles when needed, and training with compound movements when not. For this, implementing bodybuilding principles and exercises in my workout program is defiantly a must.

- Calisthenics became popular in the 21st century, as a new form of training, requiring no gym membership and using only the body's weight in order to exercise tension over the muscles. Based around compound movements executed with a set of bars, calisthenics parks started to appear, allowing more and more people to start working out without having to pay for a membership. I personally enjoy calisthenics, and a good portion of my workouts consist of bodyweight exercises, with the added benefit of being able to train at home when time doesn't allow going to a gym. Another, in my opinion very important, benefit of calisthenics, is how efficiently it burns fat, as the high amount of compound movements activate more muscles causing them to consume more calories, resulting in more rapid fat-loss.

- Crossfit has a bad rep among bodybuilders and calisthenics enthusiasts as well, and personally I can only agree with them, as crossfit trains movements rather than muscles, through a form of execution of the exercises that allows for more repetitions but with far worse quality. The tension exercised over the muscles is less than typical bodybuilding or calisthenics provide dramatically, and has the added risk of injury. I personally do not include crossfit-like workouts simply because I find them ineffective.

- Group training is the second biggest form of physical exercise in terms of popularity, and for good reason. For people looking to lose weight and gain some muscle and muscle definition, group training classes offer a less expensive alternative to a personal trainer, having a professional instruct a group of people and having them follow along through a set of explosive exercises, with energizing music and atmosphere, making the workouts fun and efficient. Some principles of group training, especially in terms of fat loss, were implemented in this book's workout program.

For the actual routine, you will have a set of bodybuilding and calisthenics exercises, with a few group training inspired cardio workouts, made simple, with little to no equipment needed. What I recommend you buy, are a set of dumbbells with adjustable weights, a set of 5kg kettle bells, and a jump rope. Without further to do, here we have the structure of the workouts.

Workout structure

In terms of exercise, there are 3 main movements, pulling, pushing and cardio, all of them playing an important role in any fitness routine. For our system, you will train 5 days a week, with workouts lasting 30-45 minutes, which you can complete in the comfort of your home.

Monday	Tuesday	Wednesday	Thursday	Friday	Saturday	Sundays
Push	Pull	Leg/Cardio	Rest	Push	Pull	

The push-pull-legs split is an advanced mechanism used by bodybuilders to be able to train the same muscles twice a week, providing the most stimulus to the muscle fibers. Having 3 days between the Push days for example provides sufficient time for the fibers to regenerate and strengthen, and the soreness to fade away.

Push days combine exercises for the muscles that rely on pushing movements in order to activate, such as the chest, triceps, and shoulders.

Pull day uses the same principle for the back and the biceps, as those muscles require the movement of pulling in order to strengthen.

Legs have specific exercises, that involve mostly pushing, but as we are talking about the lower body, having sore muscles still regenerating in the upper section of our body doesn't interfere with training the legs.

Cardio uses all sorts of exercises, based upon raising the pulse and burning calories, but with this system, cardio becomes easy.

Push Day

      The core exercise for push days are going to be pushups, which we highly suggest you master. The pushup is an amazing exercise, as it targets primarily your chest, but as secondary muscles the shoulders and triceps also get engaged, providing stability and strength in order to maximize the power output, through which process, not only does the chest grow, but so do the secondary muscles involved in the performance of this incredible exercise which military, calisthenics and bodybuilding training heavily prefers over other, more popular forms of exercises.

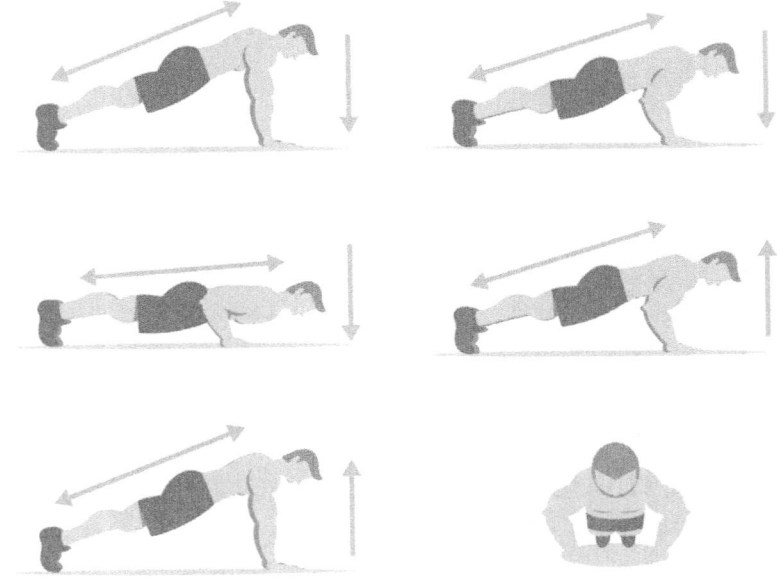

This set of images show the correct execution of the push-up, as correct form is absolutely essential with all exercises. Starting with the hands directly below the shoulders, feet back, and a straight back, the imaginary line from your feet to the shoulders should be close to 45 degrees. After getting into position, the movement is slowly lowering your body, with the elbows near the body, until you're basically parallel to the ground. The last phase of the exercise is to **push** your body away from the ground, flexing the chest and triceps, while the shoulder stabilizes.

The push-up will be the absolute core of the push-days, with different variations in order to target different areas of the body, we will use variations of the hand positioning, and the body's positioning to the ground.

First up, hand positioning, we have the classic pushup, with the hands under the shoulders, finding perfect balance between the tension over the chest, and the tension over the triceps. Next up, we have the so-called **diamond pushup,** a variation which has the hands positioned directly under the chest, with its name coming from the shape the hands make when they touch underneath the chest, primarily targeting the triceps, along with the added help of the chest. Last type of pushup based on hand positioning, we have the **wide pushup,** which, as the name suggests, has the performer position their hands about an inch or two outward, increasing the distance between them, in a wider position, this variation targets the chest primarily, keeping it under heavy tension even when the body is upward.

The second type of variation come from the positioning of our body compared to the floor. The classic pushup uses a horizontal positioning, with both the feet and hands on the ground or matt, targeting the chest in its whole, but some isolation work is typically required for an intermediate level. By having our arms or feet positioned upper than the other, we get the elevation effect which isolates either the upper or lower section of the chest. Having our feet above the hand level, by placing them on an elevated surface such as a piece of furniture, we get the **decline pushup**, focusing on the lower chest, a great exercise for isolating the lower section, while both the shoulders and triceps get engaged in one dynamic movement, without the use of expensive machines or other forms of equipment, the sheer positioning of our limbs allows for incredible methods of training.

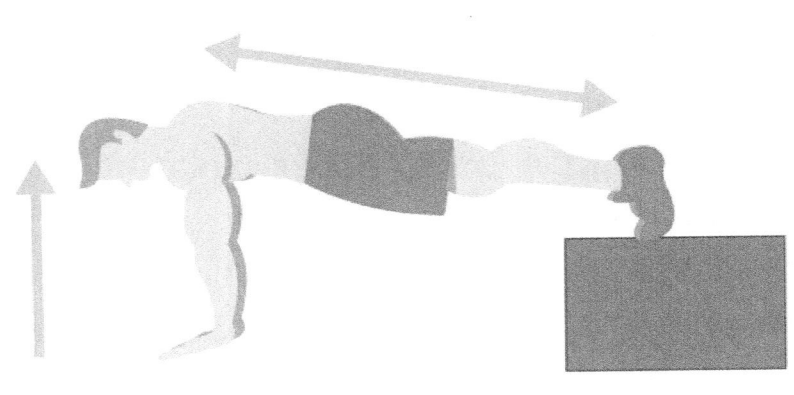

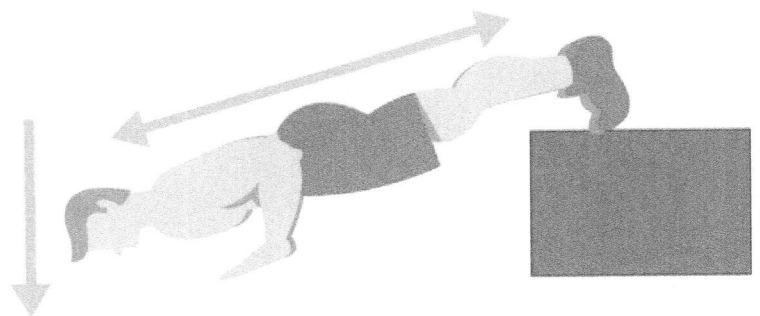

The second variation in terms of body-positioning is going to be the exact opposite of the decline pushup, by having our hands higher than our feet, we get the **incline pushup** position.

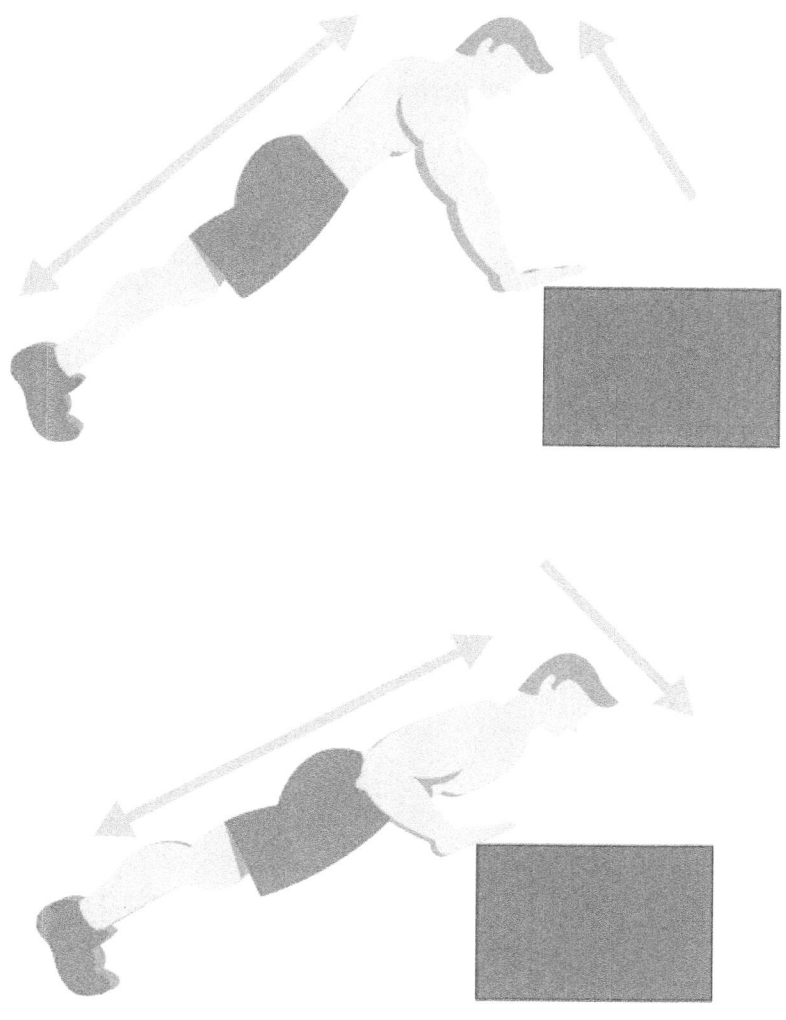

As mentioned, this is the opposite of the decline pushup, allowing for the isolation of the upper chest area, while engaging the triceps and the shoulders slightly better than the decline pushup.

The next big exercise we are going to implement is the **lateral raise,** as one of the two shoulder exercises of this routine. We only need so little since the pushup already helps build the shoulders, and push days will rely heavily on different pushup variations.

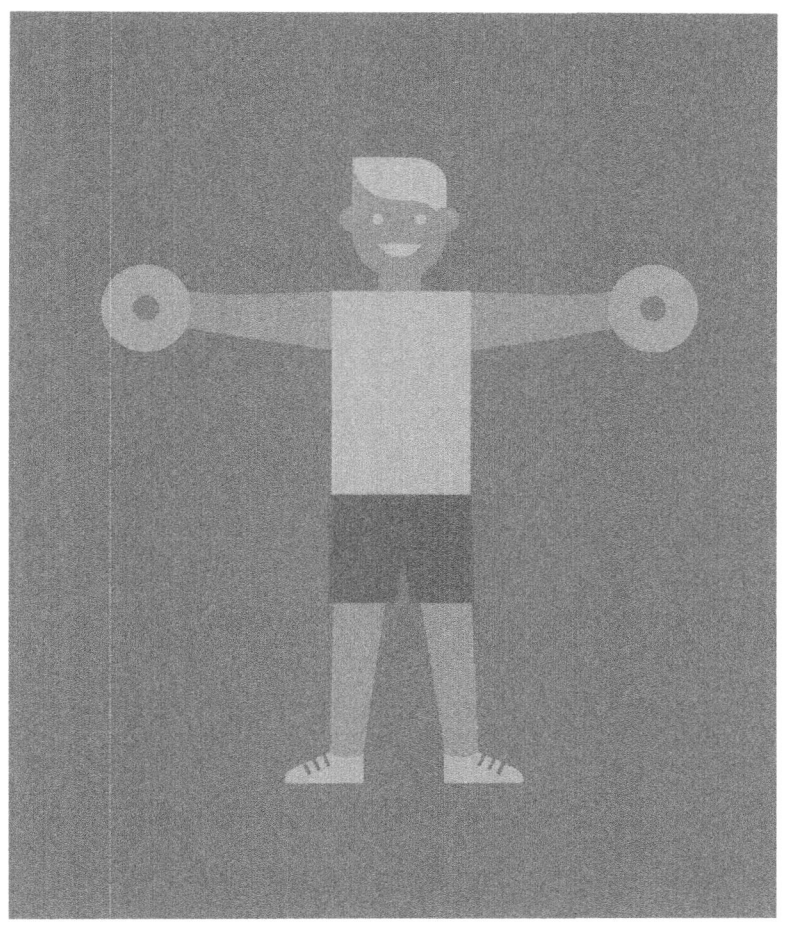

The lateral raise requires dumbbells or some sort of weights, even one gallon bottles will be sufficient in the beginning, as the shoulder's anatomy allows for great training with light weights, since the three principal parts of the shoulders fall into the "small muscle" category. The lateral raise has the one training lift the dumbbells from the side of their hips, all the way into a position that leaves the arms horizontal with the shoulders, while keeping the arms straight, or just slightly bent. Incredibly effective, the lateral raise targets the lateral deltoid in its whole, by the correct execution of the lifting movement, done **slowly**, in order to provide hypertrophy.

    The other important shoulder exercise will be the **kettle-bell shoulder press**, for which you will need either a kettle-bell or a dumbbell. The movement will have you push the weight above your shoulder, while keeping the abdomen tight, elbows slightly bent and a slow and delicate movement. It is important when building shoulders to think about the actual goal, hypertrophy, and not to push as much weight as many times as possible. Broad shoulders look fantastic on both men and women, having the separation of the shoulder from the arm creates a visual image of a V shape, helping your waist look smaller and the upper body stronger. The biggest mistake "bodybuilders" make, especially young men, is to focus entirely on isolating the shoulder, without paying attention to the actual anatomy and functions, leaving out on compound movements such as pushups. The second big mistake is to exclusively train for mass, and neglect keeping the body fat levels under control. Having broad shoulders requires a low enough body fat percentage to actually make the separation from the arms visible, otherwise the size and beauty of this amazing muscle remains invisible.

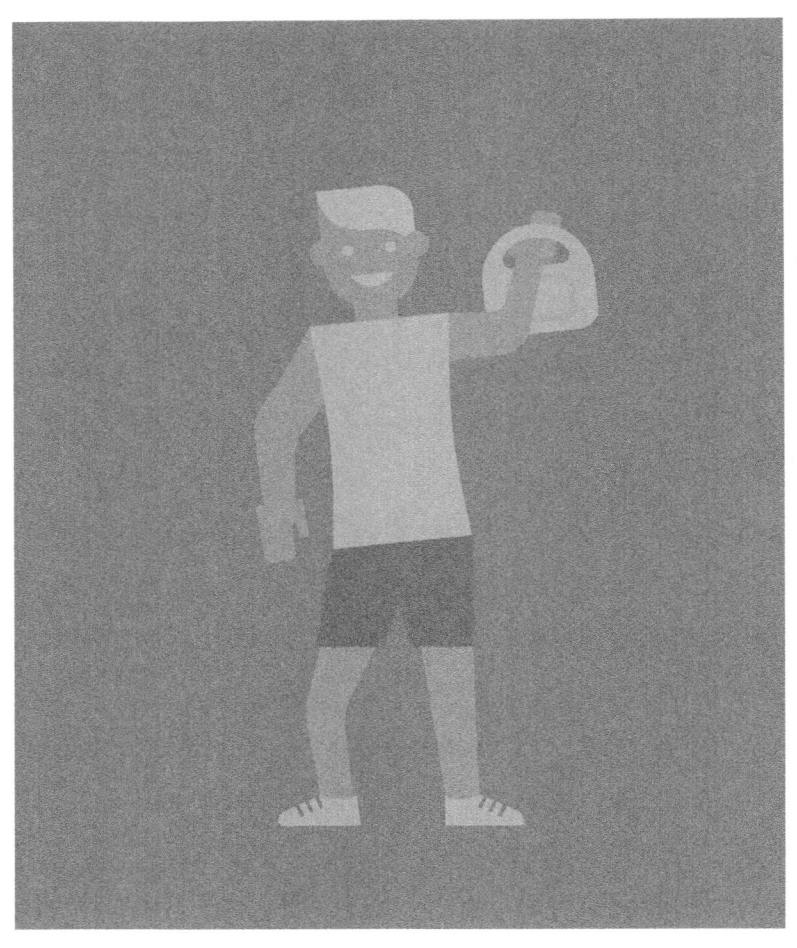

As for triceps, the amount of stress and tension we expose them to through the use of high amounts of pushups will be sufficient to ensure proportional growth and development, without having to focus on isolating the triceps completely. To further break down the push day system, heavy amounts of pushups will prioritize the growth of the chest, which is the biggest muscle group under the push day and esthetically, as a follow-up to the growth of the chest, the triceps and shoulders automatically undergo growth as well, as your body has to keep up with the development of the muscles proportionally. **Diamond pushups** have a high triceps priority, and are more than enough to grow the arms' back half. The shoulder support our body during pushups, and the tension they hold up will grow them accordingly, however, a truly good looking physique doesn't only have proportionate shoulders, in fact, the "beautiful" broad shoulders we want are out of proportion, as they are slightly bigger than the average human anatomy should have them be. For this, we added the extra shoulder exercises. The way we will schedule the workouts will follow the one above, but the two push days will not be the same, as one will focus on resistance, the other on functionality, meaning that one day will have only 1-3 exercises done abundantly, while the other will focus on more variations and more complex execution. The actual workout program will be found at the end of the book, giving you 3 workouts for the resistance push day, and 3 for the functional day, along with instructions on how to combine them and how to increase difficulty.

Pull day

Pull day is the second essential training day which will use the same system of training twice a week. For this, you may consider buying a pull-up bar for home, as the pull-up is the most important exercise in this category. Probably most readers are not capable of doing more than one or two pull-ups, which is totally fine, as it is not an easy exercise, but with time you will need to get into it. First and foremost you should start with assisted pull-ups, and make your way up from there. In order to achieve the desired results, training your back and biceps becomes most efficient through this incredible exercise.

The three exercises are going to be **pull-ups, assisted pull-ups** and **negative pull-ups.** Yes, only pull-ups. This phenomenal exercise stimulates the growth of the back muscles and biceps incredibly effectively, adding an extra bicep exercise there for extra tension and you have the perfect pull day routine. Notice how the three exercises are not only variations of the pull-up, but they are variations based on difficulty, meaning that when first starting, regular pull ups will be too difficult, so the main exercise will be the assisted one. This routine helps build strength, in order to assure the increase of performance. Not only that, but the bicep plays an essential role in executing a pull-up, thus, growth will be observed in the arm area very soon. This pull day routine is mostly based on calisthenics, as in my opinion it is the best way to build strength and back muscles.

Assisted Pull-ups will require an assistance band, you can purchase one in the closest sports store, and are quite inexpensive. Most stores offer these resistance bands in three different colors, green, yellow and red, based on how strong the elastic is. I advise starting off with a red band, as it gives the most leverage. When training, loop the band around the bar, and have your feet inserted in the other end, and having all of your bodyweight go straight down on the band, stretching it out. This will put tension on the elastic, then, holding the bar with your hands about 2 inches apart from the shoulder width, simply pull yourself up. This action engages the back and the biceps, and with the help of the band, doing 8 to 12 repetitions becomes relatively easy.

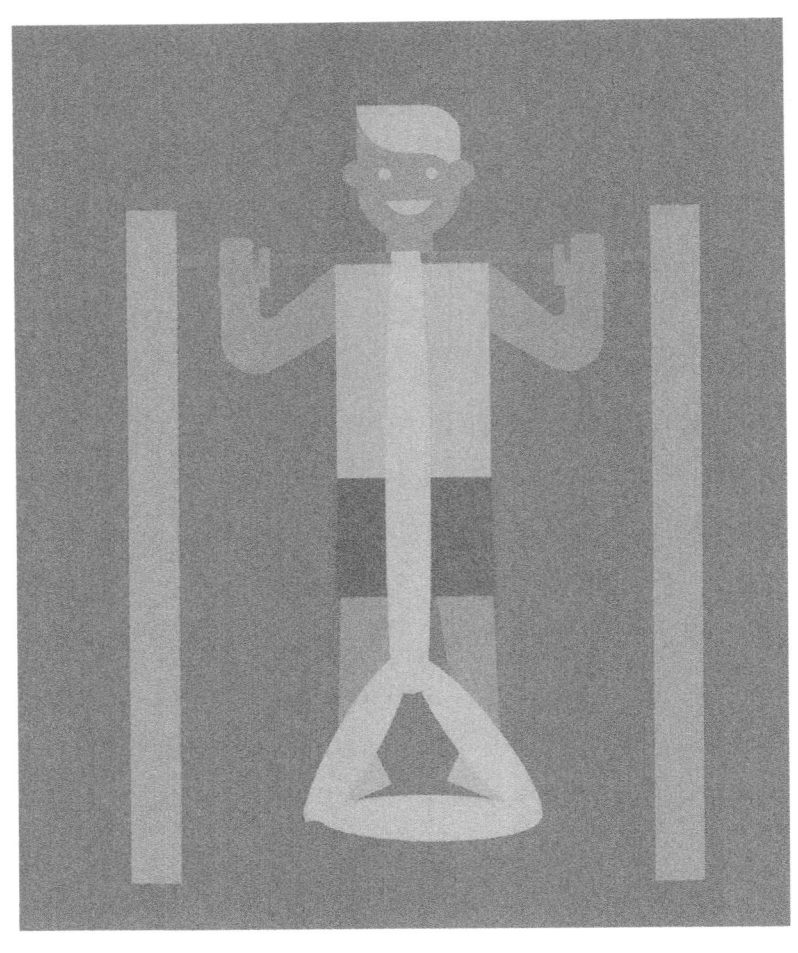

The next exercise to train your back and biceps if you are unable to do pull-ups are the **negative pull-ups,** a variation that gets around the problem of strength. By negatives in bodybuilding, we refer to having the body do the work, by keeping resistance to gravity. To simplify, the negative pull-up has you jumping to the bar and holding on to it, while letting gravity do its work and pull you down. The key here is to try to hold yourself up, fighting gravity. As you've already engaged the back muscles by jumping and grabbing the bar, you want to keep them flexed for a longer period of time, and having to hold on to the bar and slowly let yourself down keeps that tension on the muscle fibers.

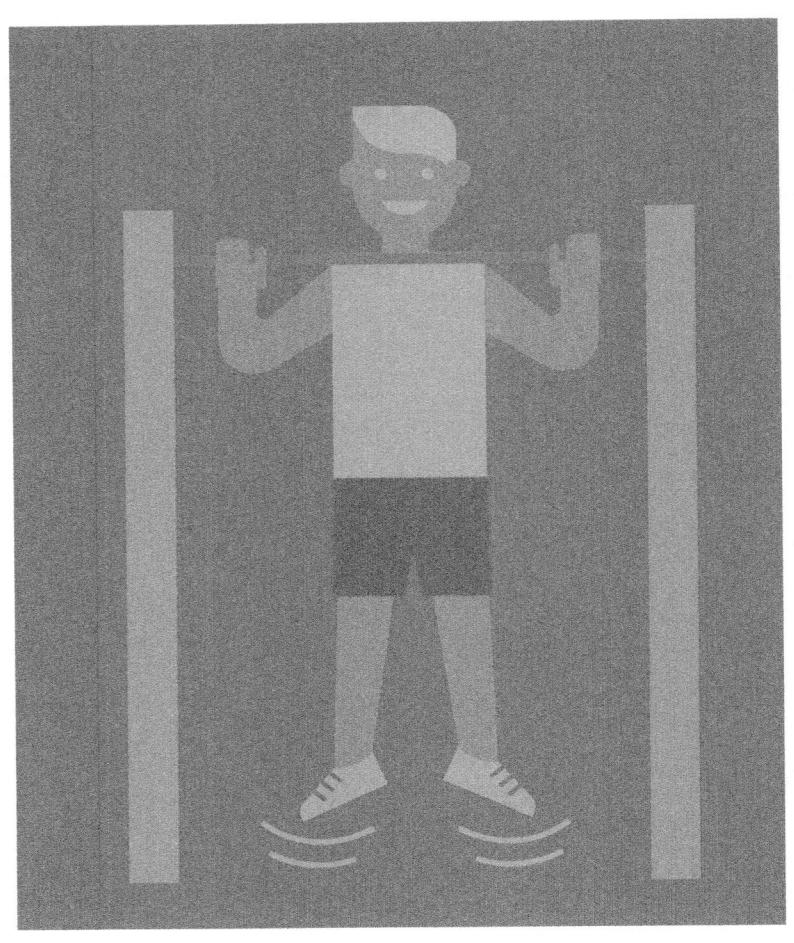

The ultimate goal with these exercises is to get your strength up, in order for you to be able to do regular pull-ups. The classic pull-up is the godfather of all back exercises, activating the back and biceps in a fantastic way, to ensure growth. Even professional bodybuilders use this exercise on a regular basis due to its incredible effectiveness. The regular pull-up is the core essence of any efficient back workout, as described in one word, this exercise is purely: **perfect**.

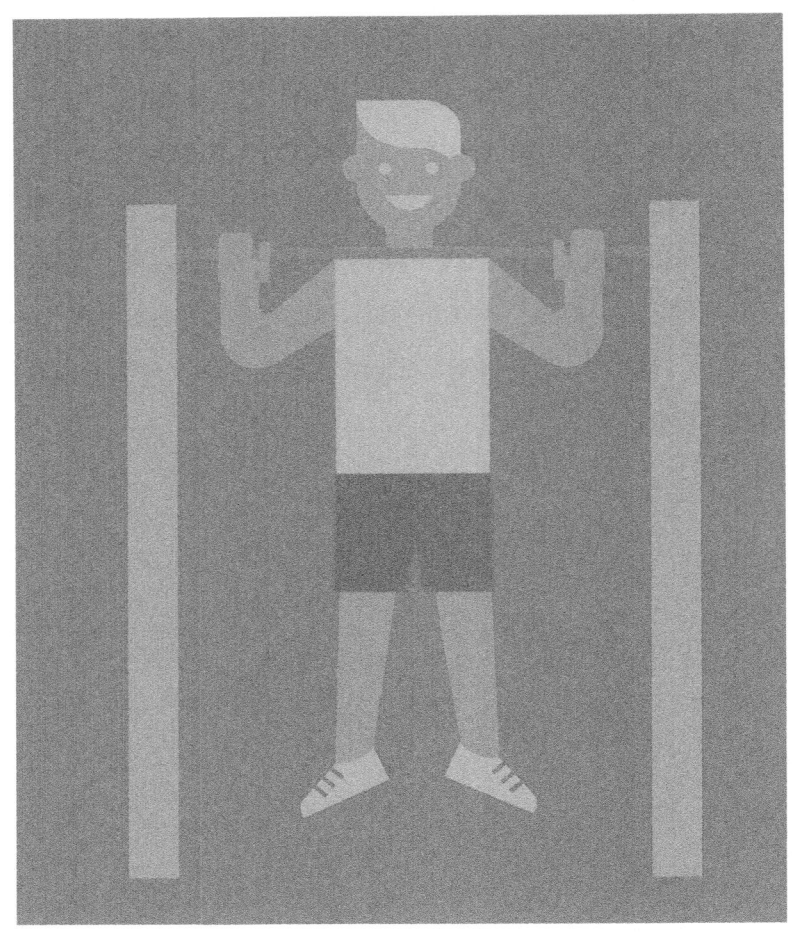

With the hands positioned as seen in the drawing above, pull-ups offer the absolute best tension and flexion of the back and bicep muscles, if the execution is correct. The main point is to get the shoulders as high as the bar, and to maintain control. Do not execute the pull-up with sudden movements, as the time spent under tension shrinks, so do the effects.

Lastly we have the bicep curl, and exercise to compliment the engagement and tension already exercised on the biceps. A dumbbell of 5-12,5 kg. is going to be recommended, but a kettlebell will work just as fine. Starting from a relaxed position, with the dumbbells in each hand, lifting the weights almost to the shoulders, in order to flex the bicep and engage both of the muscles which make up the known biceps. Arm growth is already going to be stable from the excessive pull-ups, and the bicep curl only complements this.

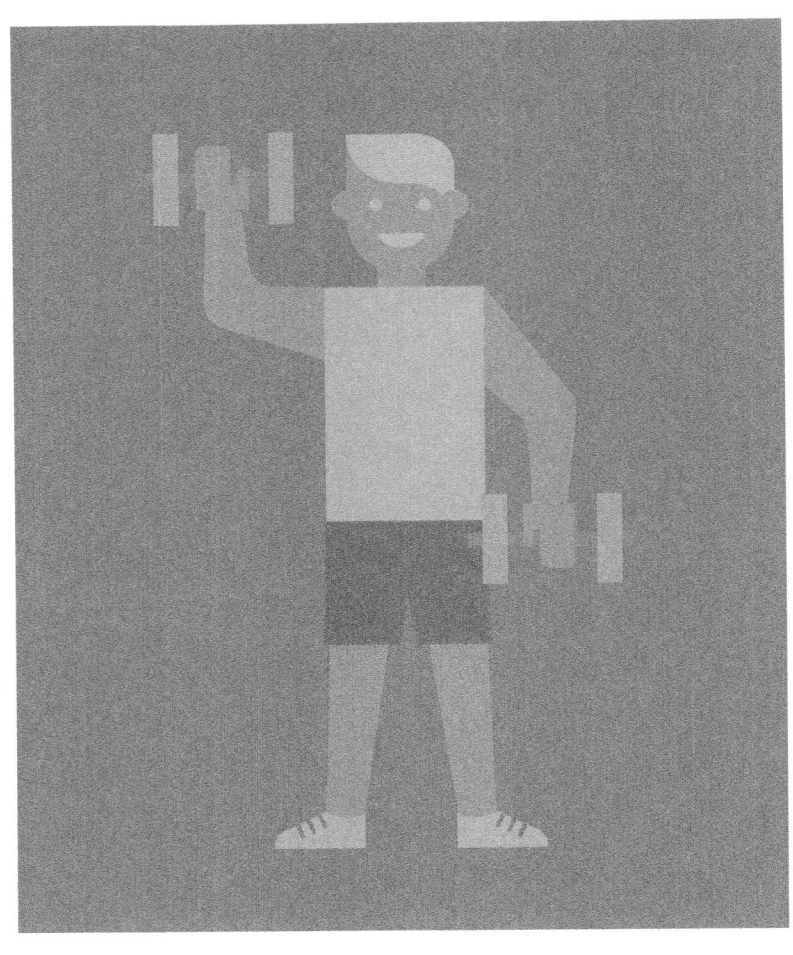

Do not forget that "big arms" don't mean only big biceps, as the actual effect of big arms is achieved mostly through the growth of the triceps. The latter make up roughly 2/3 of the arm size.

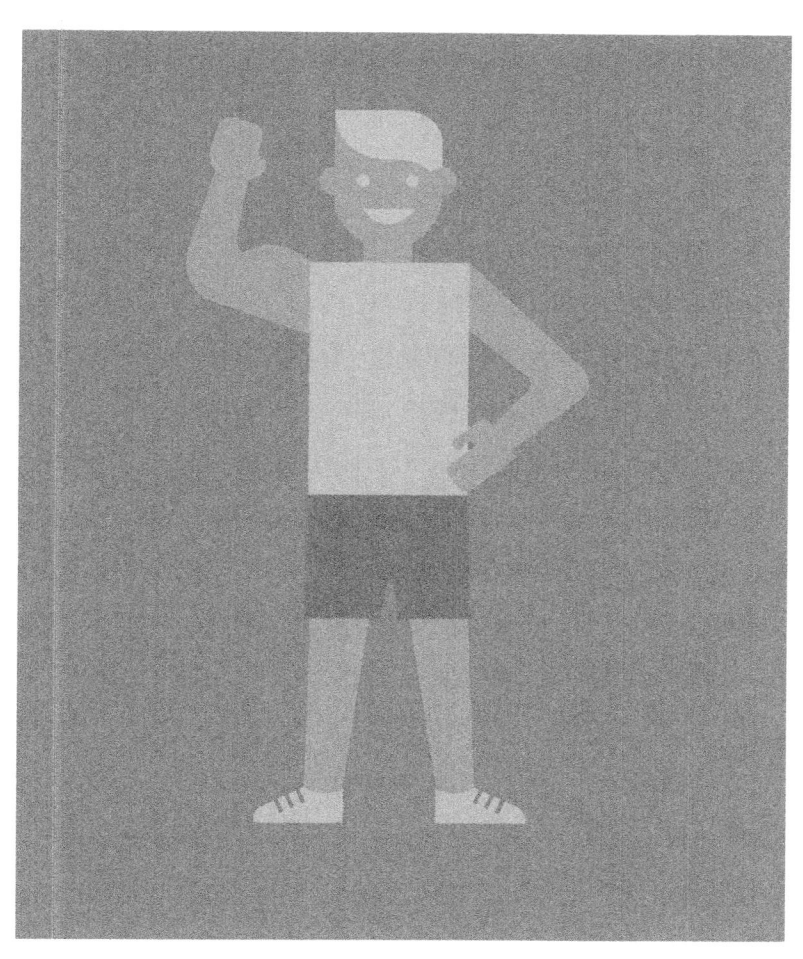

Leg Day

Probably the least liked yet mandatory training day, leg day is a must in my program as well, but in order to make it more "likeable" we only incorporate one leg day per week, and use only two exercises, the Squat and the Lunge. Keeping this simple, growing your leg muscles finds its importance when it comes to strength, calorie consumption and overall look. Some people are naturally gifted with muscular legs and strong calves, others are not. You do not need humongous quads in order to look proportionate, but a "fair" amount of muscle gives a nicer esthetic to everybody.

Starting off with the squat, this exercise is a classic, used by bodybuilders on a regular basis, activating the leg and butt muscles. Starting off with the legs positioned in shoulder-width, toes pointing forward, you slowly go down, keeping a STRAIGHT BACK and the knees from moving forward. The key to a correct squat is to go down until the lines from your knee to the ground and from your knee to your butt form a 90 degree angle. The arms can be extended for more balance, especially in the beginning, when this can mean a problem. Another essential element in the correct squat is to pay attention not to lift your heels from the ground, having all of your weight concentrated on the whole foot.

Squats can be extremely effective even with trained individuals, as a high number of repetitions can defiantly induce soreness, in time however an increase of difficulty will be required, for which, adding weights is the single best solution, instead of focusing on learning more difficult forms of this exercise such as the one legged squat.

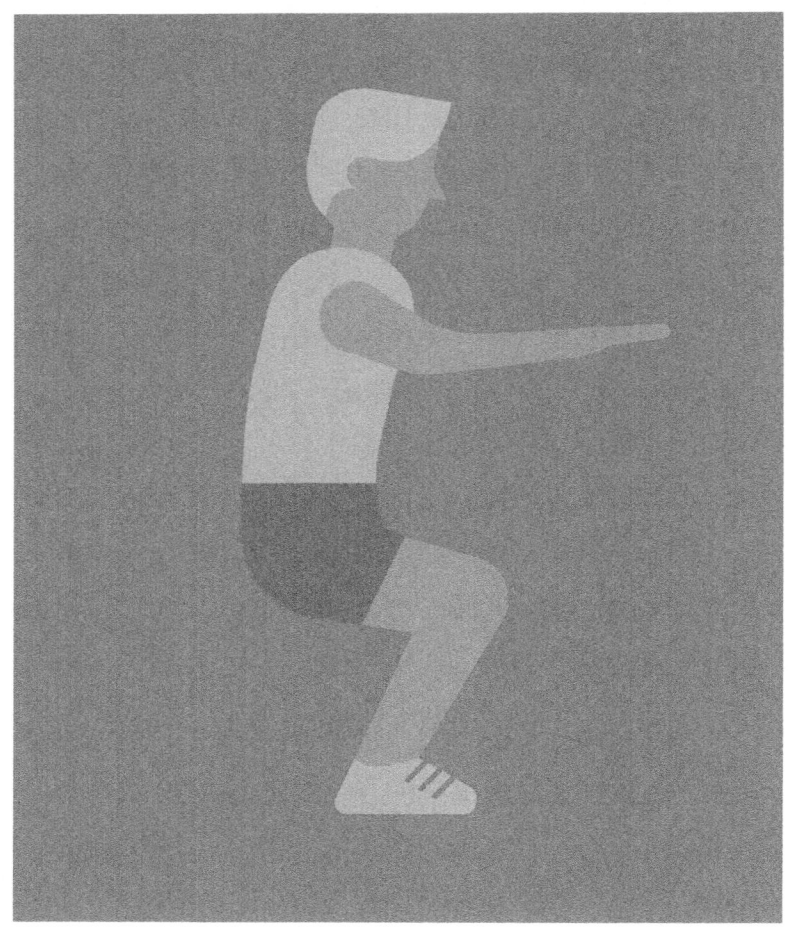

And a depiction of the squat performed with kettlebells:

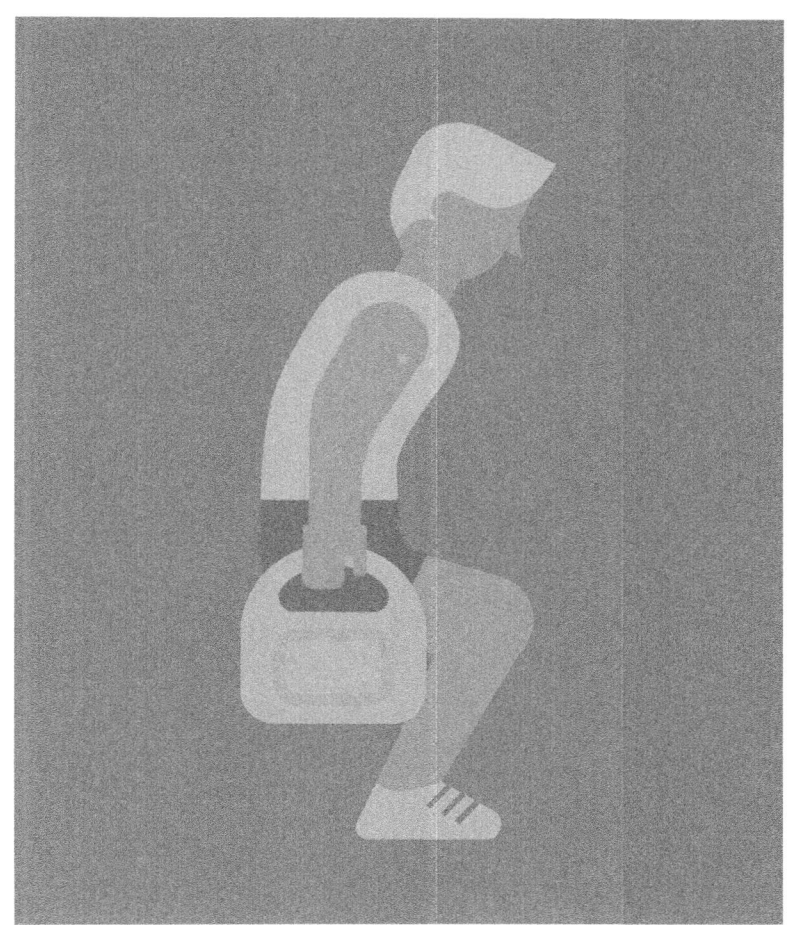

Our second exercise for the development of the leg muscles is going to be the Lunge. A more detailed video of the actual mechanics of the lunge can easily be found on the internet, but we're quite confident that most people know what the Lunge is from basic high-school sports classes. Otherwise, the lunge consists of making one big step forward, with the toes pointing in front, while having the rest of your body go down, all the way until the opposite knee touches the floor, while keeping the back straight and the legs tense.

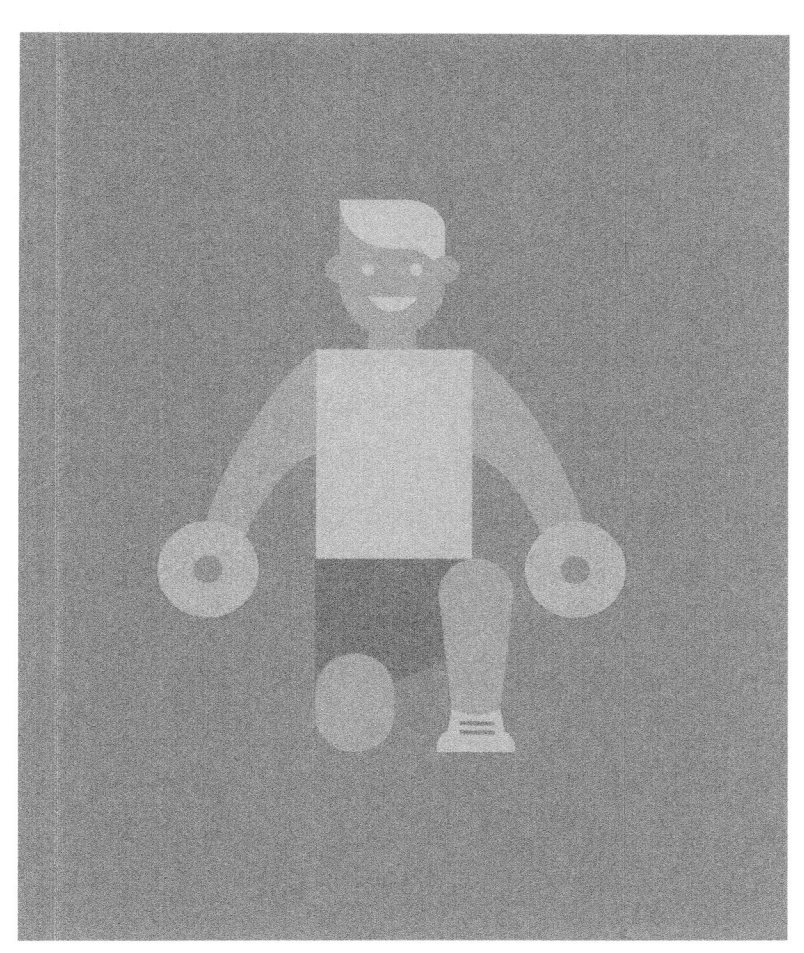

Abs and Cardio

The notoriety of chiseled abs drives more and more people to do excessive ab training chasing the 6 pack dream. In reality, having actually visible abs is a lot more simple and a lot more complicated at the same time. Training the abdominal muscles is indeed needed, in order to grow them in size, however, if the body fat percentage of the individual is too high, the freshly trained abs will not be visible. The BIGGEST mistake people make when chasing a 6 pack is to focus on training the muscle too much, while neglecting cardio and nutrition. If you want to get a hint of a six pack, or your body fat is already low, it may be enough to train the muscles and do little work towards lowering your body fat, but most often this is not the case.

We decided to structure abs and cardio under the same heading because they go hand in hand. Having strongly chiseled abs without doing cardio and paying close attention towards nutrition (the next big paragraph) is almost impossible, as the muscles grow, will result in strong abs, but the space in between those abdominal squares will be layered with body fat, making the actual progress and effort less visible.

Starting with the abs exercises, we only need two. The abdominal muscles that we want are the 6 squares to form the endlessly popular six-pack, thus we need to train all 6 muscles. The way we are going to do this is through an exercise targeting the upper and middle row of abs, and another targeting the lower and middle row, starting off first with the **sit up**, and following up with the **leg raise**.

Both will require frequent training and high numbers of repetitions, as instead of doing tens of exercises and overcomplicating your training, we keep this simple and efficient. Personally to this day whenever I'm training abs, I do roughly about 200 sit ups and 100 leg raises, as it is enough for me to feel sore the next day, especially since I do them without any breaks in between. You can train abs for 30 minutes a session, but why? The same can be achieved in 5-10 minutes of doing no break repetitions of two exercises, until total failure of the muscle is achieved. Sit ups consist of a laying position, with the knees bent and the upper body resting on the back. The repetition is the action of lifting your upper body about 45 degrees or less, in order to contract the abdominal muscles, with the arms either on the chest or along-side your torso.

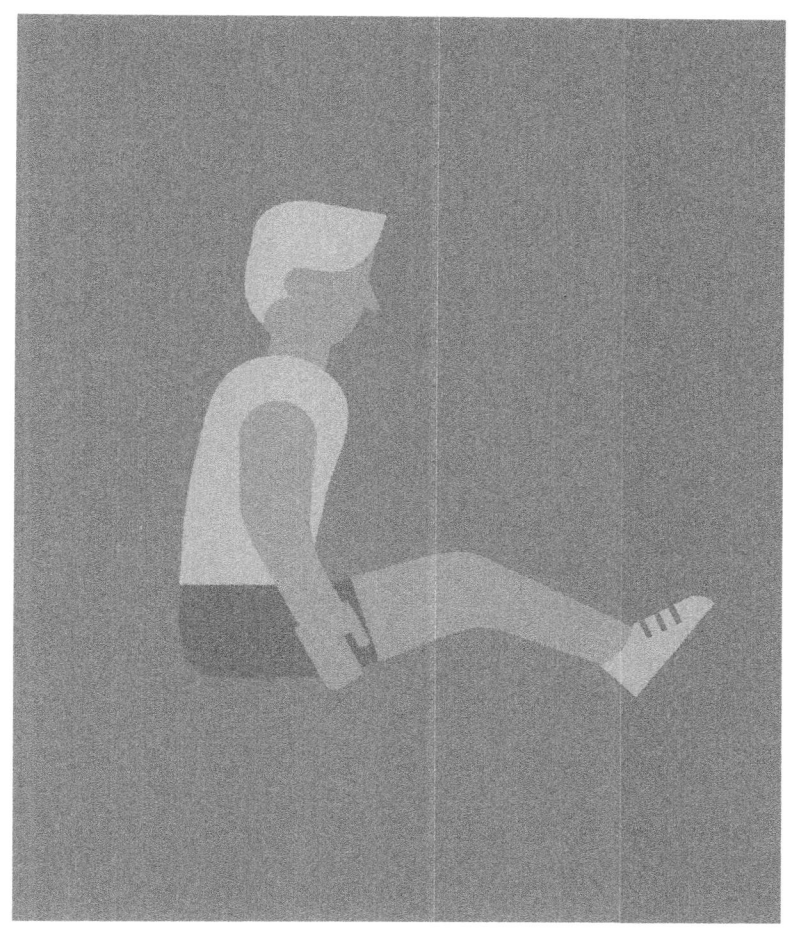

If you cannot go all the way up, no problem, the strengthening of the abdominal muscles comes in time. For the second exercise, the position is the same, laying on the back, but for this, we will be lifting our legs, 90 degrees parallel to our body. This will contract the abdominals engaging the lower row of abs.

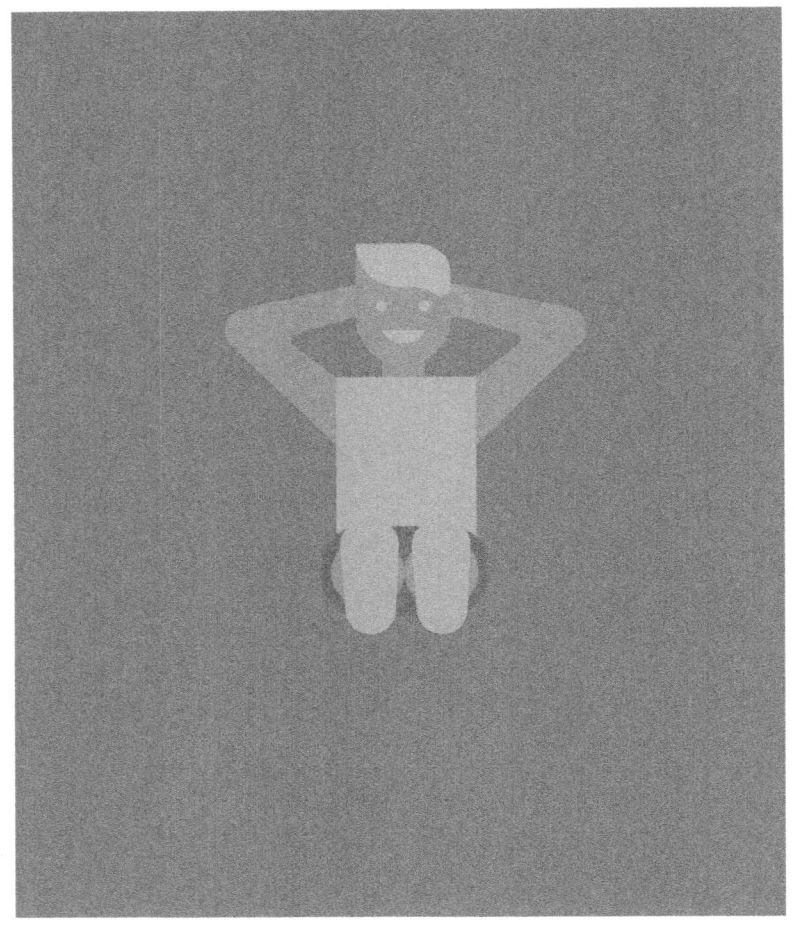

For the cardio section, I wanted to create a system that is both efficient and doesn't require excessive amount of miles ran or exhaustion. For that, I chose to implement the system I used for the past year to shred body fat, doing 10 minutes of cardio for 6 days, and one session of running the last day. Obviously, for the beginning these numbers will change, with the optimum probably being 2 days with 10 minute quick workouts and one day with a more difficult running session.

For the first exercise, we have **knee taps** or knee raises, whichever name you prefer.

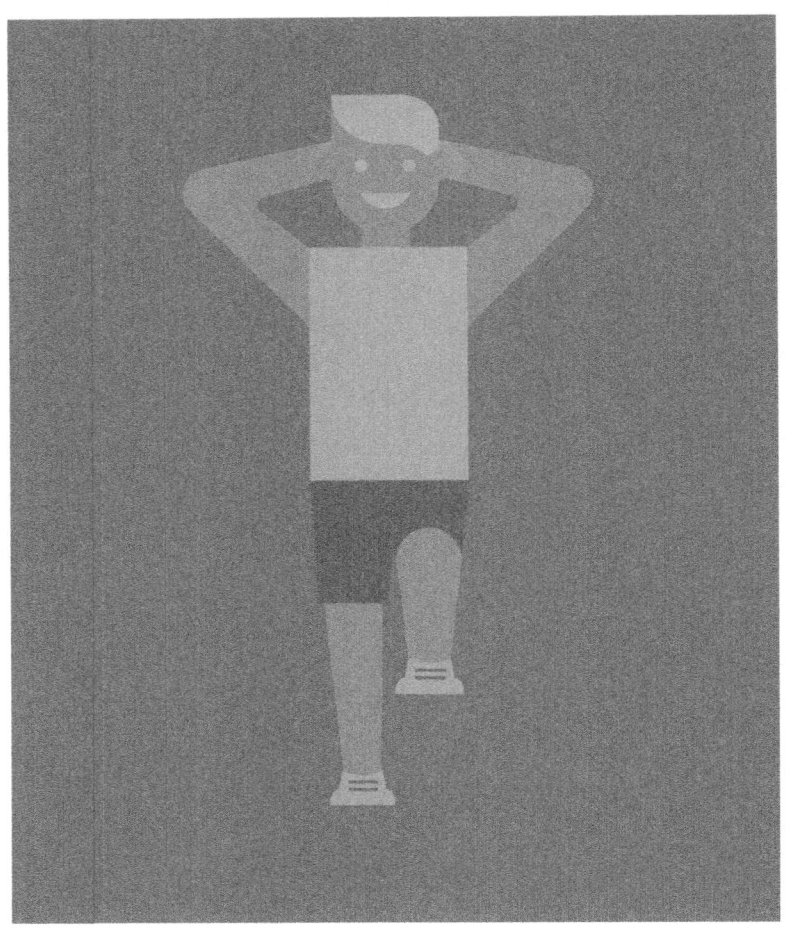

Extremely simple, this consists of having the hands on the back of your head or along-side the torso, and running in place, with the knees raised up. We will talk about how much to do and how at the end of the book when we talk about workout programs. For now, it is sufficient to know that this is going to be your fat-burning best friend.

Lastly we have **running**, which doesn't need much of an explanation at all.

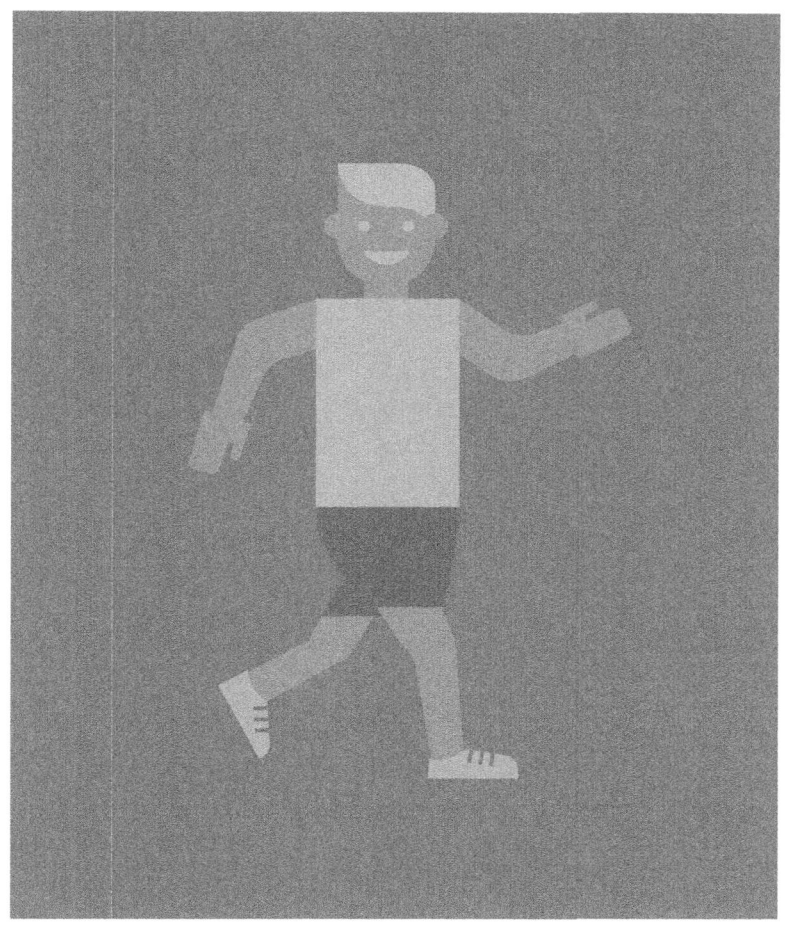

As an alternative to **knee raises**, I bring you one of my all-time favorite exercises, **jump rope**. Whenever you see boxers training with this exercise, know that it is not only for the sake of cinematography, as jump rope is an amazing way to burn fat and increase resistance and endurance. If you are willing to train the actual movement, as it can be difficult for someone unfamiliar with jumping rope, I highly recommend switching the knee raises with jump rope.

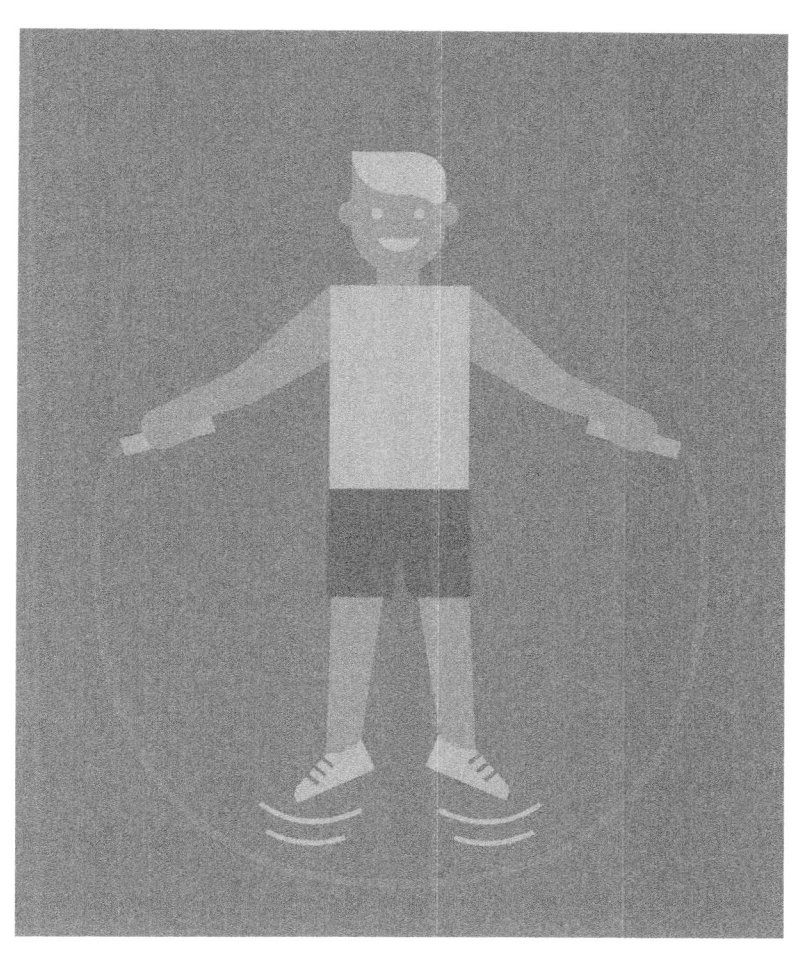

Nutrition

The second pillar of an amazing body is the nutrition plan we follow. For the beginning we need to get rid of "toxic" food and replace them with healthy alternatives which are less caloric. Then, we will focus on an eating schedule, and we will use the only one I find effective, intermittent fasting. I've been following this plan for the past two years, and the results after the first 6 months were amazing, and I highly recommend trying an intermittent fasting system to all of my elderly clients, as it helps combat the slowing metabolic rate we experience after the age of 40.

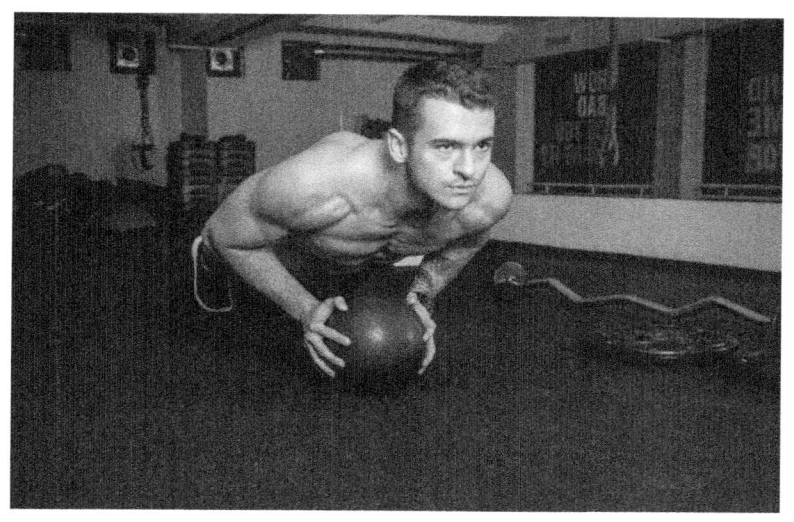

I have never had the striations on the chest and the veins on the shoulders visible before, so I stand proudly on the side of intermittent fasting, which spread widely across the fitness community and for very good reason. I included the full guide on how to get started with this system along with a basic nutritional instruction page.

If you are unfamiliar with the concept of intermittent fasting we'll go over it in short, then we will be looking at the basics about nutrition, and after that, we're getting into the amazing benefits and system of intermittent fasting, allowing for a diet without as many restrictions, but still promoting fat-loss and muscle gain, as well as saving you time and money.

Intermittent fasting is the nutritional schedule based on intentionally fasting yourself, for a period of time, then later consume as much food as you want in your eating-window. This revolutionary method allows for guaranteed weight loss over a short period of time, while not restricting the variety of foods you can eat. Just how and why intermittent fasting works, what are its benefits and why should you use this phenomenal way to diet in order to achieve the best visible results fastest? These are the questions we'll answer, including some tips to make sure your intermittent fasting goes easily and smoothly, without having to deal with cravings outside your eating window.

So how does intermittent fasting work? First of all, before heading into the basic fasting technique and schedule, you will need to understand how weight loss and gain work, from a strictly scientific point of view.

No new revolutionary weight loss method works based on magical supplements or techniques, it's all based on the science of physiognomy. Intermittent fasting does work better than other diets or strategies, but it's all in the simple logic people tend to look past.

The Basics

Nutrition is key to any fitness program. Your body is capable of amazing things, just think about how our body grows and develops in the first 18 years of our life. We are born with only a few pounds, yet, we rapidly develop stronger muscles, our bones grow and strengthen, our whole organism adapts to new challenges. In order to achieve this, however, our body requires certain resources. Humans are omnivore, yet we do need certain vitamins and minerals found only in meat, vegetables, fruits, grains, which, in the XXI. century, we can supplement. One thing to remember is, that no supplement can compete with actual healthy food.

The correlation between eating and gaining / losing weight takes place when it comes to our caloric rate.

Most people are familiar with the calorie / kilocalorie measurements, the scientific definition is: *"A calorie or calory (archaic) is a unit of energy. Various definitions exist but fall into two broad categories. The first, the small calorie (symbol: cal), is defined as the amount of heat energy needed to raise the temperature of one gram of water by one degree Celsius at a pressure of one atmosphere. The second, the large calorie or kilocalorie (symbols: Cal, kcal), also known as the food calorie and similar names, is defined as the heat energy required to raise the temperature of one kilogram (rather than a gram) of water by one degree Celsius. It is equal to 1,000 small calories."*

Our bodies require a certain amount of calories daily, in order to live a healthy life. This number varies from person to person, depending on aspects such as sex, height, weight, age. There are many formulas for calculating our needed caloric intake, the simplest and best option would be to go online and search for " calories calculator ", and fill out an online formula. For people who would like to calculate it themselves, we'll recommend the World Health Organization's 1980 equation.

Formula :

Females: Age 3 to 9 years = 22.5 x (Weight in kg) + 499 Age 10 to 17 years = 12.2 x (Weight in kg) + 746 Age 18 to 29 years = 14.7 x (Weight in kg) + 496 Age 30 to 60 years = 8.7 x (Weight in kg) + 829 Age over 60 years = 10.5 x (Weight in kg) + 596

Males: Age 3 to 9 years = 22.7 x (Weight in kg) + 495 Age 10 to 17 years = 17.5 x (Weight in kg) + 651 Age 18 to 29 years = 15.3 x (Weight in kg) + 679 Age 30 to 60 years = 11.6 x (Weight in kg) + 879 Age over 60 years = 13.5 x (Weight in kg) + 487

Let's say you are a 22 year old female. The average American woman over the age of 20 weighs 168.5 pounds and stands at just above 5 feet 3 inches. Based on this information, by introducing this data into an online calorie intake calculator, assuming you have a sedentary lifestyle with little to no exercise, we'll find out that you need 1,789 calories a day, this number will vary based on your lifestyle activity, that's why we recommend using an online calorie calculator to accurately determine how many you actually need. This number shows how many calories you have to take in, in order to maintain your weight.

Obviously things change when you are a 52 year old male, looking to make an improvement in their physique, that's why we included the formulas for all age groups, so you can accurately calculate the amount of calories needed to be taken in.

The basic principle of weight gain and loss is simple, you eat less calories than you need, you lose weight, you eat more calories than needed, you gain weight.

Notice we said "you lose weight", not fat. Indeed by eating less calories than you need, you will lose fat, but also muscle. This is why usually an exercise program is recommended when we are trying to lose fat, not only it speeds up the process, but it maintains our muscle mass, and help lose as much fat as possible, while losing as little to no muscle. Another thing worth noting is that we use the term "nutrition", not "diet". The reason behind this is that most fit people, consider eating healthy a lifestyle, while a diet is something you do for a determined period of time.

In the following, we will focus on how to apply these rules, in order to lose fat, depending on your determination and expectations. As we said, you can skip exercising and still lose weight, with a significant part of it being fat. However, if your goal is to get those abs to show, maybe thicken those arms as a male, or tone your legs and butt as a female, in order to look your best this summer, exercise and a more strict approach to your nutrition will be required.

You can find how many calories are in every food on the back of the package, or online. Based on that and using a kitchen scale, you can determine how many calories you took in with every meal. There are countless calorie tracking apps to download to your phone, instead of writing down every meal. We suggest using an app as it makes it a lot easier to keep track of your daily and weekly calories.

Before we dive into the actual nutrition plans, depending on how determined you are, first let's take a look at some foods you should automatically avoid if you are looking to lose weight. These foods are high in calories, have little vitamins and minerals, and are best avoided or substituted for their low-calorie, diet-friendly alternatives.

Soda – any type of beverage, with the exception of water, tea, coffee should be avoided. Also we recommend having tea or coffee with no sugar, or, with artificial sweeteners, like Stevia. The substitute for these drinks would be their 0 sugar versions, which are more unhealthy but have little to no calories.

Pasta – go for whole grain pasta or rice noodles.

Pastry – extremely packed with carbohydrates and calories, not fulfilling, pastry should not touch your plate or mouth if you are aiming for a summer body.

Sweets – anything that falls into the category of desserts, candy, or treats, will be considered an enemy. You can find 0 sugar chocolate and candy in most supermarkets, usually sweetened with Stevia. Also we will cover many delicious treats for you to eat, that will not harm your physique.

Fast food – another pretty obvious category, no burgers, fires, fried chicken, tacos, or anything you can get at a drive-through should be consumed. Most of the food you eat should be made at home, or, if you are eating out, go for a restaurant, not a fast food place.

Deep fried foods – Anything fried in a bunch of oil, from fired chicken to French fries. Their healthy alternatives will be food cooked in the oven, with a little bit of olive oil, and sweet potato fires, made in the oven.

White bread – Replace white bread with whole grain or an even better alternative for a slice of bread would be a rice cake.

White rice – Replace with brown rice.

Alcohol – All alcohol should go, in case you want to have a drink with a special occasion, blonde beer, white wine and gin are the least caloric alcoholic drinks.

Just by giving up on these foods, you could lose a few pounds in a relatively short period of time. A former high school friend lost more than 40 pounds over the course of about 5 months just by giving up on soda, sweets, and bread.

Having sorted out foods that will surely stop you from losing weight, here are a few quick snacks to munch on, whenever you get the cravings.

- A handful of nuts (literally as much as you can fit in one hand)
- Protein shakes (in your desired flavor)
- Popcorn (few calories)
- Greek yoghurt with **fresh** fruits
- Fruits (excluding grapes and pears for their high sugar content)
- Sugar-free candy
- Protein bars
- Oatmeal
- Rice cakes with orange slices
- Dark chocolate (1-2 squares)

Having given you some general information about foods to avoid and foods to try, now let's go into more detail about how to apply this information in order to lose weight / fat, based on your level of dedication.

The easy way

The most basic weight loss technique, has only one requirement, consume less calories than you need. While it is widely debated what that number should be, a sure spot would be about 400 to 500 calories less, daily. So if based on your data, you should eat 1800 calories, aim for eating only 1300 – 1400.

Using a kitchen scale to track the amount of food and calories it contains, going on a caloric deficit is scientifically proven to make you lose weight, based on how the human body works. This way however, you will end up losing fat as well as muscle.

Since we are not looking to overly complicate things for our readers, by eliminating the foods we listed to avoid, and switching for their healthier counterparts, combined with calorie tracking to get to a caloric deficit of 400-500 kcal, you should be good to go. However, we do recommend taking the harder approach, exercising and eating a specific set of foods we'll list in the next section, in order to truly unlock that body you always wanted.

As mentioned in the beginning, the real way to lose fat and build a better body is combining nutrition and exercise, first thing's first, you will be eating healthy food. Completely avoid the foods listed in that category, and focus on eating mostly high quality products. Using your kitchen scale, measure your meals and calculate their caloric data.

As we dive deeper into nutrition, you'll have to understand that food is made up of 3 main macro-nutrients. These are fats, carbohydrates and proteins. The most important one of the 3, from a fitness point of view, is protein. Protein is necessary in order to build and maintain muscle, and usually, more protein-rich foods are also lower in calories.

The base of any weight loss program:

- A slight caloric deficit (aprox. 200 kcal)
- Protein-rich foods
- Quality foods
- Lots of vegetables
- Water (hydration)

- A few tips and tricks listed at the end of this section

Since we are trying to make this whole program as easy as possible for you, we are going to list certain food ideas, for each meal of the day. You are going to be eating 3 main meals and 2 snacks.

Breakfast: Protein, Carbohydrate, Fruit

Lunch: Protein, Carbohydrate, Fruit or Vegetable

Dinner: Protein, Carbohydrate, Vegetable

Snack 1: Fruit

Snack 2: One of the snacks listed bellow

Protein ideas:

1. Chicken breast
2. Chicken drumstick
3. Tuna
4. Lean beef
5. Lean pork
6. Cottage cheese
7. Eggs (super-food)
8. Whey protein powder
9. Home-made shake (we'll get to this)

Carbohydrate ideas:

1. Brown rice
2. Wholegrain bread
3. Sweet potato
4. Oatmeal
5. Beans

Fruit ideas: You can have pretty much any fruit, however we do recommend avoiding grapes and plums, when it comes to fruits, your serving should be 1 piece. 1 banana, 1 orange, 1 apple, etc.

Vegetables: Try avoiding regular potatoes, other than that, you can have other veggies in any quantity.

Snacks:

1. Handful of nuts

2. 2 rice cakes with thin layer of honey and cinnamon

3. Greek yoghurt with <u>fresh</u> berries

4. 2 teaspoons of peanut butter

5. 2 squares of dark chocolate

6. 2 handfuls of popcorn

7. 5 low calorie biscuits

These will be your principal ingredients, since we don't want to overcomplicate things for you, here is a diagram of how you should proportionate your food. Half of your plate should be filled with veggies, a quarter with protein, and another quarter with carbohydrates.

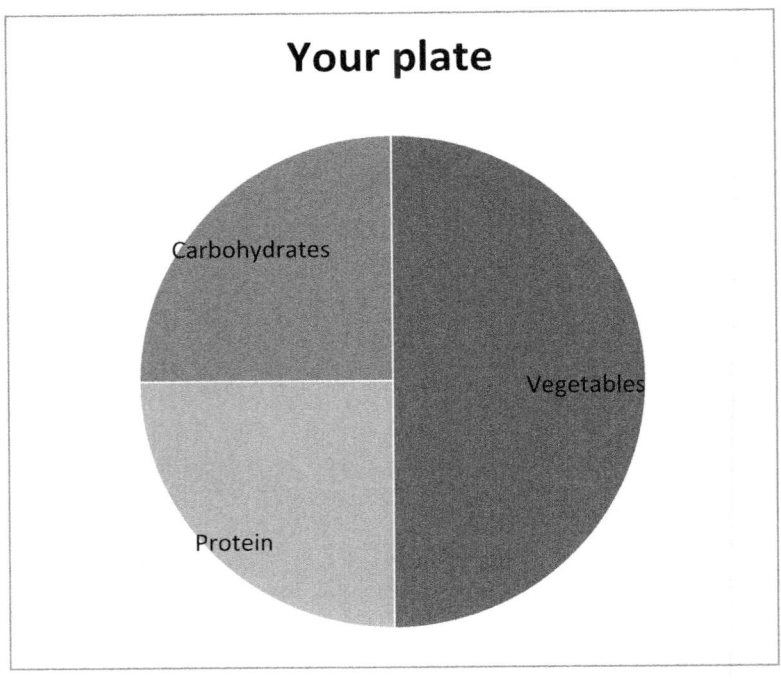

This is essentially all the general information you need to know about nutrition in order to achieve fat-loss. Further we'll discuss some tips and tricks we've found really useful, don't forget, results aren't achieved by doing just a few big things, it's also the small things that add up.

Tips and Tricks

- Cinnamon can help burn fat. Eating 1-2 teaspoons of cinnamon a day will help you in burning fat, obviously you are not supposed to eat it by itself, you can spread it through your meals and coffee. A teaspoon of cinnamon in your morning coffee, 1 in your Greek yoghurt and you are all set.

- Having a banana or other fruit before working out will increase your energy levels drastically.

- Drinking 3L of water a day. It may seem much, but if you set a goal for yourself, like drinking a 1L bottle during your workout, 1L from morning to noon and 1 more liter spread out through the day, it is not even that difficult.

- Going to sleep early will reduce the risk of late-night cravings.

- Drink a glass of water before every meal, and before going to sleep.

Intermittent Fasting

Now that you've gained some basic knowledge on how our bodies' weight loss / gain systems function, we ask the question, "So how and why does intermittent fasting work?"

Intermittent fasting allows more flexibility to your diet, as it's not as restrictive as the basic diet structure presented above, giving you the chance to munch on all your favorite foods in your eating window. But not to debunk the biggest myth surrounding intermittent fasting, it's not the actual fasting that works magic.

There are 3 main structures to the fasting program:

Alternate day fasting - 24/24 1:1

This fasting type is by far the most difficult to follow, as it requires you to go a full day without eating, then allows 1 full day of eating freely. This cycle repeats for as long as you can repeat it, but the main drawback here is the necessity to control your hunger a full day, which can make daily tasks difficult, due to lack of energy. This is especially determinant when it comes to people who work out. As you could've read in the section explaining nutrition and weight loss, exercise plays a huge role in any body-shaping goal, and working out without eating for a full day can be very challenging and even start catabolism, the process of breaking down muscle fibers in order to produce energy. Of course, there is the possibility of training during the days you are not required to fast, but that can lead to inconsistency in training, especially for those who work out 5 times a week.

Day 1	Day 2	Day 3	Day 4	Day 5	Day 6	Day 7
Day 8	Day 9	Day 10	Day 11	Day 12	Day 13	Day 14
Day 15	Day 16	Day 17	Day 18	Day 19	Day 20	Day 21
Day 22	Day 23	Day 24	Day 25	Day 26	Day 27	Day 28
Day 29	Day 30	Day 31				

Fasting	Eating

5 : 2 Fasting

The second fasting program is taking things a bit lighter, yet is probably the least effective in terms of weight loss. This principle uses 5 days of normal eating and 2 days of fasting, which, in real terms is not all that relevant.

Day 1	Day 2	Day 3	Day 4	Day 5	Day 6	Day 7

Fasting	Eating

While it still requires you to go 2 full days without eating, the remaining 5 days are more than enough to overrun the caloric deficit made during those 2 days.

The 16 : 8 intermittent fasting ratio

Probably the best fasting regime both in terms of difficulty and effectiveness has its focus on fasting periods over a day, rather than over weeks or months. Meaning that instead of having full days for fasting and full days for eating, it gives the advantage of being able to eat every day, while still fasting daily. The structure of this system is going 16 hours fasted and 8 eating.

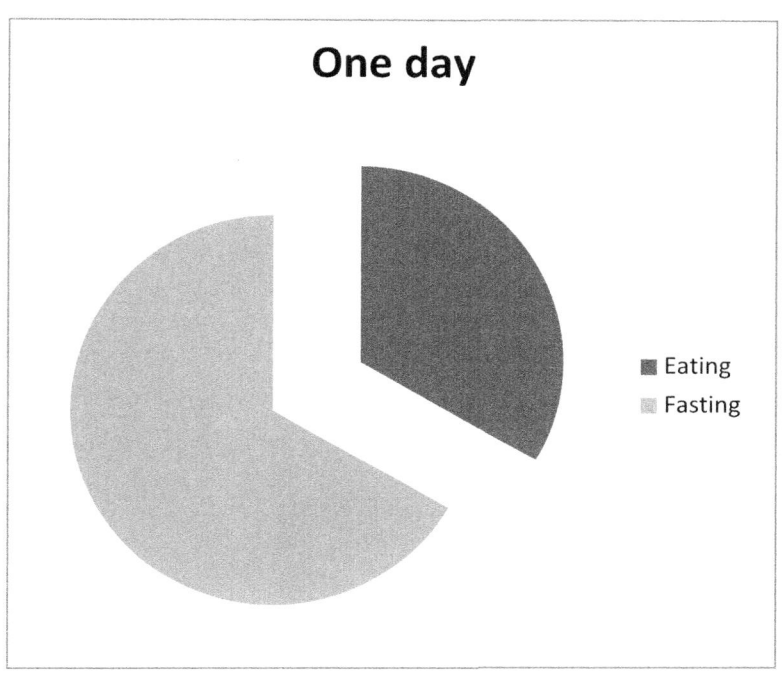

In terms of difficulty, the 16 : 8 regime is most advantageous since you don't have to go days with no food, yet, it's the easiest out of very difficult ones. By no means intermittent fasting will be easy to achieve for everyone, that's why further we'll also take a look at some tips and tricks to use when fasting, to make it easier for you to go with this fasting technique and achieve the desired weight loss.

As for effectiveness, this program allows training every day, since during the 8 hour eating window, you can fill up on energy, and get kicking in the gym, while the 16 hour fasting period is enough to directly activate the weight loss functions.

Getting started

When you first start intermittent fasting, you should have the last meal of that day at 20:00, this way your fasting-eating schedule starts at a time that will make it the most convenient to live with. Now you won't be allowed to eat until 12:00 the next day, right around noon. From noon to 20:00, you are in your eating window, so this is the time interval for eating all the food you get that day.

At first, it will be difficult to go from waking up to 12:00 without eating a single bite, the only things you are allowed to consume are water, tea, and black coffee, obviously with no sugar or sweeteners. We say black coffee since milk does have calories and falls in the category of food, thus stopping your fast.

Also a difficult part of fasting will be having craving after 20:00, since you're outside the eating window, and is the most common time for munchies.

Before we break down the science behind Intermittent Fasting, let's go over some tips to make it as easy as possible to fast without feeling the constant need to eat.

The main idea behind making Intermittent Fasting work, is to make you feel fuller for a longer period of time, and there are certain nutrients that highly promote that, as well as few small tricks to avoid getting the cravings.

#1. Get proper sleep

One of the reasons why teenagers and young adults tend to be fat, or should we say more fat than the previous generations is lack of sleep. Sleep is strongly believed by scientists to be linked with the levels of ghrelin and leptin hormones. Lack of sleep increases the levels of ghrelin, the hormone responsible for the feeling of hunger, while also decreasing leptin, the hormone which promotes the sensation of fullness.

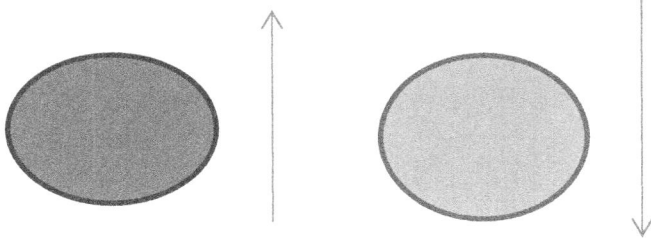

The combination of these actions greatly affects any weight loss program or binge eating control, so tonight maybe skip one or two episodes of your favorite Netflix series, and end the group chat earlier, because the recommended sleep duration is 8 hours, in order to control hunger and decrease binge eating.

Studies concluded that sleeping less than 8 hours per night is strongly linked to higher bodyweight.

With all that being said, by going to sleep earlier, you automatically exclude the chance of eating more, and will end up spending 8-10 hours of your 16 hour fasting period asleep.

#2. Increase protein intake

Protein and fiber are both scientifically proven to help with bodyweight and cravings related problems, so let's look at both separately.

Protein is the most precious nutrient for bodybuilders and fitness enthusiasts, and for good reason. It's the main nutrient associated with muscle gain, increased metabolism, and promoting fullness. A study which had their subjects increase their protein intake by 15% not only showed decreased bodyweight and fat mass, but also a reduced daily calorie intake, by an average of 440 calories.

Some common protein rich foods are eggs, tuna, chicken breast, protein shakes and fish, all of them are great for any weight loss program.

#3. Eating more fiber

Fiber moves slowly through your digestive tract, making you feel full for longer. Fiber is just pure magic when it comes to cutting craving, reducing bingeing and calorie intake, as it makes us feel fuller, and for a longer period of time, and countless studies back this up. The best thing about fiber is how inexpensive it is, fruits, vegetables, whole grains, all of them are packed with fiber, but possibly the best option when it comes to this superstar of foods, is oatmeal. Oatmeal is super cheap, and can be prepared in a variety of ways, depending on your personal preference, form protein oats to fruit oats, it's completely up to you.

#4. Drink more water

Hydrating yourself is probably the simplest yet most effective way to overcome hunger and cravings. A variety of reasons is present behind this claim, firstly the physical aspect, if you drink more water, you eat less. By filling your stomach with water, less room is available for food, and it works every time. If you want to prove it for yourself, before your next meal, drink 500ml of water, and see how much will you eat, compared to the usual.

Studies show that increased water intake can be linked to weight loss and reduced cravings, as one study conducted on 30 adults, showed that by giving them 500ml of water before eating, they consumed 13% less calories than the group that didn't have water.

Athletes consume more water than the average person, for the highly possible benefits on their physique and performance. Other studies show that water intake can be related to boosting your metabolism, which, along with its fulfilling effect, can make up a significant part of your hunger suppressing process.

Why exactly does intermittent fasting work?

Well, as nutritional and medical professionals will say, the weight loss does not happen due to the actual fasting period, or because of any undergoing effects that occur due to fasting, the reason is a lot more simple.

The reason why most people lose weight while fasting, although they eat regular food, with no restrictions lies in the eating window itself. It becomes fairly difficult to eat more calories than your daily needs, when you have to consume them in under 8 hours.

Studies show that subjects that were following intermittent fasting, ate fewer calories than their daily needs, thus a constant caloric deficit was born. A caloric deficit results in weight loss anyhow, but may be more difficult to achieve if allowed to eat all day 'round.

In conclusion, Intermittent Fasting relies on programming its followers to eat in an 8 hour window, in which case, it become highly probable that they won't eat in a caloric surplus, but rather in deficit, added that most subject will try to also follow a healthier alimentation while fasting, the results are pretty much guaranteed.

There is a catch however, even if you do go with intermittent fasting, but during the given 8 hour window consume highly caloric foods, and manage to eat over your caloric needs, weight gain is going to appear. The probability of this situation occurring is fairly low, so as long as you try to restrict yourself to eating somewhat healthier foods, while still consuming your favorite treats in a reasonable amount, you're good to go!

Rest

As for the rest section, as essential as recovery is, there is not that much to talk about. In the essence, you need a solid 8 hours of sleep every night in order to be sure that your muscle cells regenerate bigger and stronger.

When dealing with soreness, do not forget that a muscle group takes up to 2 days to recover, after that, even if you are sore, it's safe to train. The best way to cure soreness is through training, as the first set will feel terrible, due to muscle pain from the soreness, the next set will feel amazing, as the first one cures the soreness.

Training plan

Now that we've discussed the exercises, the diet and a bit about rest, it's time to move on to the most important part of this book, the workouts themselves. First, we'll give you examples of workouts for each day, then, we will move on to structuring those sessions into a 7 day cycle.

Push days

E1	Exercise	Repetitions	Sets
First	Push up	8-12	4-5
Second	Incline Push up	10	4
Third	Diamond Push up	8	5
Forth	Decline Push up	10	3

This is the first push day workout, on the first column, we have the order of the exercises, and we do as it follows, first we do 4 to 5 sets of 8 to 12 push-ups. After the 4-5 sets are done, we move on to 4 sets of 10 incline push-ups, etcetera. The "E1" in the corner stands for Easy 1, as it is the first workout of the Easy push day ones.

E2	Exercise	Repetitions	Sets
First	Push up	16	4-5
Second	Wide Push up	12	4
Third	Incline Push up	10	5
Forth	Diamond Push up	8	3

M1	Exercise	Repetitions	Sets
First	Push up	20	5
Second	Incline Push up	15	4
Third	Wide Push up	16	4
Forth	Decline Push up	10	5
Fifth	Diamond Push up	8	3

Sixth	Lateral Raise	24	3

M2	Exercise	Repetitions	Sets
First	Push up	25	4
Second	Wide Push up	16	5
Third	Lateral Raise	12	4
Forth	Incline Push up	10	5
Fifth	Shoulder press	12	5
Sixth	Diamond Push up	8	5

H1	Exercise	Repetitions	Sets
First	Push up	MAX	5
Second	Incline Push up	MAX	4
Third	Decline Push up	MAX	4
Forth	Wide Push up	12	5
Fifth	Diamond	12	5

	Push up		
Sixth	Lateral Raise	20	6

H2	Exercise	Repetitions	Sets
First	Push up	MAX	5
Second	Wide Push up	MAX	4
Third	Diamond Push up	MAX	4
Forth	Wide Push up	12	5
Fifth	Diamond Push up	12	5
Sixth	Lateral Raise	20	6

U	Exercise	Repetitions	Sets
First	Push up	MAX	4
Second	Incline Push up	MAX	4
Third	Decline Push up	MAX	4
Forth	Wide Push up	MAX	4

Fifth	Diamond Push up	MAX	4
Sixth	Lateral Raise	MAX	4

Pull days

E1	Exercise	Repetitions	Sets
First	Assisted Pull up	10	6
Second	Negative Pull up	8	4
Third	Bicep Curl	12 / arm	5

E2	Exercise	Repetitions	Sets
First	Negative Pull up	6	6
Second	Assisted Pull up	12	5
Third	Bicep Curl	12 / arm	6

M1	Exercise	Repetitions	Sets
First	Pull up	6-8	4
Second	Assisted Pull up	16	5

Third	Negative Pull up	8	4
Forth	Bicep Curl	12 / arm	5

M2	Exercise	Repetitions	Sets
First	Pull up	6-8	4
Second	Assisted Pull up	16	4
Third	Negative Pull up	10	5
Forth	Bicep Curl	12 / arm	5

H1	Exercise	Repetitions	Sets
First	Pull up	MAX	4
Second	Assisted Pull up	20	4
Third	Negative Pull up	10	4
Forth	Bicep Curl	MAX / arm	3

H2	Exercise	Repetitions	Sets
First	Pull up	MAX	4
Second	Assisted Pull up	MAX	4
Third	Negative	8	4

	Pull up		
Forth	Bicep Curl	MAX / arm	3

Leg day

E	Exercise	Repetitions	Sets
First	Squat	12	4
Second	Lunges	10 / leg	4
Third	Squat	12	3

M	Exercise	Repetitions	Sets
First	Squat	25	4
Second	Lunges	16 / leg	4
Third	Squat	10	5

H	Exercise	Repetitions	Sets
First	Squat	40	5
Second	Lunges	20 / leg	4
Third	Squat	10	3

Cardio

Light	Exercise	Repetitions	Sets

	Jump Rope / Knee taps	60	8 - 12

Hard	Exercise	Repetitions	Sets
	Running	1 hour	1

Abs

	Exercise	Repetitions	Sets
First	Sit ups	MAX	2
Second	Leg Raises	MAX	2

And now to break things down a little, wherever we say MAX, it refers to the maximum number of repetitions you can physically do before failure.

Cardio days are inserted preferably in the morning of another training day, preferably push or pull. We do not advise doing cardio and legs on the same day. Abs can be inserted during the same day as any other workout, most efficiently after you are done with a pull, push, or legs routine, go into doing abs.

Weekly schedule

Monday	Tuesday	Wednesday	Thursday	Friday	Saturday	Sunday
Cardio light	Pull	Rest	Cardio light	Abs	Legs	Cardio hard
Push	Abs		Push	Pull		

Insert any workout in the weekly schedule you prefer, and increase the difficulty. Whenever you find the E workouts too easy but the M too hard, just increase the number of repetitions on the E until you are able of doing an M.

Printed in Great Britain
by Amazon

81798067R00068